I0412069

Raw Milk
the legal "Anabolic Steroid" for common-sense Californians!

Jumper Publications and Media
from Advice to Results

Disclaimer

The purpose of this book is to empower the reader with knowledge, to educate, informational purposes. This book is not medical advice, but rather the author's personal experience, and is a guide for anyone who wishes to implement said dietary or lifestyle changes at the reader's own discretion. The choice between medical care and self care is completely up to the reader. If you have a medical problem, seek medical care. The author and Jumper Publications and Media shall not be held responsible or liable for any and all damages, loss, or injury, of any kind that may be caused or allegedly caused, directly or indirectly, by the information in this book. Reading beyond this page is the reader's consent to the above disclaimer.

Other Publications

ABC Water and the Number Crunch Diet
a step by step solution to alkaline deficiency and
with a New and Unique approach to weight control

Nontoxic Teeth Whitening and Dental Hygiene System
"Spare me the chemicals, I've switched to FOOD GRADE to
whiten, gargle and brush."

JPM Oral Hygiene Protocol
stop using toxic drugstore mouthwash, discover how to reduce
your gum pocket depth from 3-4-3 to 1-2-1 mm when they probe

12 Changes A Year – Volume 1
the recipe book to the Number Crunch Diet
When you take control of the numbers
you take control of your weight.

NCD Flaxseed Shake Recipe
the Number Crunch Diet method for getting omega 3s
and with three variations so you'll never get bored

The 5 Points of Posture
the missing link to fat loss, overall wellness, and
to becoming Respected, Adored, and Wealthy

12 Changes A Year – Volume 2
the recipe book to the Number Crunch Diet
Begin today and forever be in control of the numbers you're eating.

To purchase additional copies, please visit

http://www.CreateSpace.com/5339343

CONTENTS

Edits & Format

You will notice oddities in punctuation, spelling, syntax, and perhaps even semantics, within this book. Feel free to let me know, but some of it is done for brevity or to shift emphasis. I use capitals where I see fit, to grab your attention and make it stand out, and I also remove capitals when I don't think they are deserving of them, or to remove emphasis after first usage, i.e., Pyrex becomes pyrex. And french bread, brussels sprouts, and english cucumbers, are spelled lowercase, as we are not going to "link" a European vacation to our food and eating.

Secondly, I will unhyphenated to create rhythm. Grammatically, two or more words that function as an adjective before a noun are supposed to be hyphenated. That's fine. A million-dollar smile, is the adjective "million-dollar" describing the smile. However, this can get redundant after a while, 1&2 3, 1&2 3, 1&2 3. The noun gets all the attention. But what if you want the adjectives to have the emphasis? After all, the adjectives are the descriptive words. So, I will drop the hyphens to allow the adjectives equal emphasis, and to change the pace of the sentence a bit. So if there are no hyphens, read it slower and evenly, one two three four five six seven. A "step-by-step solution" sounds a bit skippy and simplistic, whereas, a "step by step solution" is said slower and sounds more methodical. Hyphenating two words, or joining two words as a compound word, reduces their individual meanings.

With regard to fastfood, healthfood, and seasalt, it's time for these words to evolve into compound words, so the trend starts here.

There are also some fragmented sentences, subject-verb disagreements, and singular/plural violations. When "correcting" certain of these sentences, they lost their emphasis and punch, so I kept them as is.

In the past I've been guilty of judging other author's sentences, only to reread it with the commas, pauses, and then it made perfect sense. So, if there's a comma, then pause, as you may not get to pause later in the sentence. If there's no comma, then don't pause and read it all as one.

I pose questions, but without question marks. Some are rhetorical, but some are to make you Ponder. Great word. Ponder. If you see a question mark at the end, then it requires an answer. If there's no question mark, then you can just say, yeah, no, or hm.

English continues to change, people using it, customize the language to fit what they want to communicate, emphasize, and to make their point from various angles. It also has to have a variety of melodies and rhythms to keep it from being boring. If you find yourself having to reread a sentence, it may be that it's structured that way for that very reason. So take your time. Don't rush. Let the words digest, so that you absorb the material, and hopefully take some of it and make it a part of your life.

Lastly, you will notice that I customized the headers of every page! This is not something Microsoft Word Starter allows you to do. You can only customize three pages, first, even, and odd. So, to get around this I had to create a Page Break every three pages, and as a result, the last line of some of the pages doesn't "justify" to the edge. So I hope that flipping through the upper corners of the pages will assist you in finding the chapter that you are looking for.

You won't see any citations from scientific studies or PubMed, because at JPM we look to a higher source for our reference.

God Bless!

Enjoy the Journey

Email me if you have a question, or if you just want to comment. Your purchase comes with 3-months free support and photos.

Barry Ogston, B.Sc., CLS, MLS(ASCP)

You have to crunch the numbers to see what you're really eating.

CHAPTER 1

The Facts

Welcome.

This is an introductory booklet published by Jumper Publications.

ABC Water and the Number Crunch Diet
"A jumper is a device that connects one wire on a circuit board to another wire on a circuit board, allowing for – The Transfer of Information from One to the Other."

You will see references to other publications within this booklet, don't be upset, you paid $3 if you bought the kindle version, or $5 for the paperback version, equal to a gallon of gas or a ventimocha.

The information in JPM books you will not hear anywhere else. It's all original content. The things in *The 5 Points of Posture* you will not hear anywhere, and the Alkalinity component to your health is completely hidden in the mainstream, more popular in the alternative-health arena, but no one covers the subject as accurately and comprehensively as in ABC Water™.

So, to begin, we first need a bit of history on why raw milk was legal for centuries and then it became illegal in the 1940s, and is still illegal in most states, all of Canada, and other places, but "poor" people in underdeveloped nations are still free to drink raw milk, without their government telling them that they can't.

1   The Facts

Almost makes you wonder who's really free.

35-million Canadians are not allowed to drink raw milk because their government is looking at the wrong facts.

Fact #1
The issue isn't Raw Milk vs Pasteurized Milk, the issue is Clean Milk vs Dirty Milk.

Prior to the 1940s milk pasteurizing was not common, Chicago was the first to make it a law in 1908, but generally, it became the norm in the 1940s.

So, what was the reason for this shift?

Dirty Dairies. In Britain it was a big problem. So, dairy farms were getting sloppy in the U.S. and the solution was pasteurization.

News Flash – pasteurization is not removing the bad bacteria.

Fact #2
Dirty dairy milk means that cow butt bacteria is getting in the milk.

Now, I could say, pathogenic disease-causing bacteria, such as *Salmonella*, *Shigella*, *Yersinia*, *Listeria monocytogenes*, *Campylobacter jejuni*, *Staphylococcus aureus*, and *Escherichia coli* from the animal's stool is getting into the milk and causing illness and death in the immune compromised and elderly.

But, I'll just keep it simple and say, Cow Butt Bacteria.

As a microbiologist, not only can I spell those bacteria, I know how to pronounce them and what they look like under a microscope.

So man's solution is never as good as God's original design.

Sorry "man", you're not as smart as the Creator God. But man sure thinks he is, and so he keeps trying.

So, God's way is organic small-farm dairies, and man's way is dirty large-farm factories. So man deviates from God's ways and creates problems. Then, rather than recognizing the error of his ways, he then comes up with an idea to fix the problem, and so man drifts further away from God's design.

If you haven't read any of the other publications by JPM, we are not "religious" but we are pro-God.

Hybridization is normal, you select certain plants over others. Genetic Modification of plants and animals by inserting DNA from one species into the DNA of another species is cross-species genetic manipulation, this is man playing God.

God created the species, and there's no need to improve on God.

Common sense is another way of saying God's ways. Many people still have this. Many people have completely lost it. Hence, we have two sides of people in today's world, those who follow God's common-sense ways, and the opposition, the people who hate truth.

Fact #3
No amount of pasteurization will REMOVE the bad bacteria.

The bad bacteria are still there, they're just nonviable (dead).

So, you are eating dead cow-butt bacteria.

Fact #4
When I first started drinking raw milk from Organic Pastures Dairy Farm in Fresno, California, www.organicpastures.com, I read their entire website. I recall reading that they had never had a positive test for a pathogenic bacteria. Not one *E. coli* or bad bacteria ever in their milk, ever. Okay, I said, it's clean milk.

Then I read where the founder/owner of the dairy farm created a mobile milking machine so that he can milk the cows out in the field and not in a barn or a pen. Wow. Innovate. I'm impressed.

Fact #5
Wound bacteria is also found in factory milk. God created the cow to produce about 1-3 gallons of milk a day, and now the factories are pumping as much as 5-6 times this a day from the cow, three times as much production as in the 1960s. So this excessive milking creates wounds. The tissue dies and flesh-eating *Staphylococcus* and *Pseudomonas* infect the tissue, along with tons of cow white blood cells. Pus. There's Pus in this milk.

If you have lactose intolerance you need to rethink your intolerance. It's not the lactose sugar that you are reacting to, it's the dead cow-butt bacteria and wound bacteria and cow WBCs.

Page 276 *ABC Water and the Number Crunch Diet*, "If your mother gave you milk as an infant, which every newborn baby had, then you had the lactase enzyme when you were born. Your DNA worked then. If your DNA worked then, why wouldn't it work today?"

CHAPTER 2

The 3 Ways

Well most people won't have an answer to that last question, but the "experts" will say, "Your DNA gets turned off as you get older." Well, true, DNA can fall asleep when it's not been active for a while. It's like going hiking when you haven't gone hiking in years, those muscles were asleep. Same for your DNA. The DNA is still there and can make lactase, but you just have to wake it up.

I had this issue, as I was reacting to dairy, so I stopped drinking milk, my lactase DNA went asleep, and I became "lactose intolerant".

So I created the NCD Lactose Intolerance Protocol™, page 277.

And I went from "lactose intolerant" to drinking dozens of gallons of "dangerous" raw milk each year. I knew my DNA could make lactase, and I'll bet yours can too.

Note: The NCD Lactose Intolerance Protocol is not about drinking raw milk. This protocol is copyrighted by JPM and found in *ABC Water and the Number Crunch Diet*.

Page 321, "If you have any gastrointestinal problem, in my opinion, raw milk will fix it, or at the very least, make it less of a problem. The 'danger' of raw milk is that it could eliminate your need for pills and scopes."

Every dairy farmer knows that raw milk is a source of good bacteria, beneficial bacteria, your body's normal flora.

FYI, microbiologists use the word "flora" when referring to populations of bacteria. Botanists don't own this word.

Let's test your knowledge.

Yesterday I bought a gallon of raw whole milk at Lassen's, my local healthfood store, and it was reduced in price from $14.99 per gallon to $7.99 per gallon due to the fact that it was going to expire at midnight.

What happens to raw milk when it passes its expiration date?

Tick tock tick tock tick tock tick tock....

Buttermilk.

And what do we know about Buttermilk?

Tick tick tick tick....

It's better for you than milk because it has more beneficial bacteria.

When I opened the cap on my gallon of raw milk that was going to expire at midnight, there was a creamy layer on the inside of the cap and it had a sweet-sour smell, a bit like sour cream or ricotta cheese.

I drank half the gallon that day and the other half earlier today.

And not only did I not get sick and die, but the exact opposite happened.

MY MUSCLES PUMPED UP, I FELT 25 YEARS OLD AGAIN, AND Grrrrrrrrr!   That grab-a-table-and-throw-it-across-the-room feeling. TESTOSTERONE SURGE!

Lats expanding under my arms, delts broadening, biceps and triceps filling up, quads getting heavy and big, full body expansion, and I hadn't even worked out yet.

Now, imagine the effects when you follow raw whole milk with weightlifting. Yeah, I think you get it ('steroid-like' growth).

I drink raw milk three different ways.

1. NCD Flaxseed Shake™
See the publication *12 Changes A Year*, the recipe book to the Number Crunch Diet. This 46-page recipe was extracted from this book and published as the stand-alone book, the *NCD Flaxseed Shake Recipe*.

2. Diluted 50/50 with raw skim milk, to create raw 2% milk.

3. Consumed as is, raw whole milk, 4% milkfat.

All three ways create an anabolic effect. The degree of this effect varies from time to time, whether I've worked out or not, and which way I am drinking it, (pre-, post-, or with-workout).

Part of it is the fact that the milk is loaded with raw nutrition, unheated raw milk protein, and it's liquid, so it goes into the body fast. However, the macros are also key to creating an anabolic effect.

On the website www.abcwaterandthenumbercrunchdiet.com, you will see a photo of the NCD Taco Salad™, aka, "Anabolic" Taco Salad.

Many of the meals on the Number Crunch Diet create an anabolic effect, and I believe it has to do with the ratio of the macros of the meals, the macronutrient percents.

This is why all the meal photos that you see on the site, and that are found in the recipe books, *12 Changes A Year, Volumes 1, 2, 3,*

have identical percent macros. And calories. This is the other key.
They all have identical calories.

So going back to our "spoiled" raw milk that gets better as it ages
due to the replication of the good bacteria and the absence of cow-
butt bacteria and wound bacteria, what happens to regular store-
bought milk, say, a gallon of pasteurized milk from Safeway, what
happens to that milk when it expires?

Well, we all know, Don't Drink It. It's spoiled, real spoiled.
Throw it away. And it smells when you open it and pour it down
the drain. This milk does not turn into buttermilk. This milk turns
into garbage.

From the factory, this milk had passed the cutoff limit for bad
bacteria, but it wasn't completely free of bad bacteria.
Pasteurization kills most of the bad bacteria, and most of the good
bacteria, but then as it sits on the shelf, and the days go by, the bad
bacteria multiply and take over.

This is why anti-bacterial soaps and sanitizers are a bad idea. They
kill the good and the bad, but not all of the bad, and then the bad
multiply and take over. See the JPM Nontoxic Hand Sanitizer™
protocol in *Nontoxic Teeth Whitening and Dental Hygiene System*.

And, Triclosan, the chemical in antibacterial soap, has recently
been reported as cancer causing, liver damaging, and all the rest.

So, milk is good for bodybuilding, but if you drink dirty
pasteurized milk from your standard everyday supermarket, you
don't get the anabolic effect because your immune system is being
activated on a low level, subclinically. You're getting some good,
but you're also getting some bad, so the net result is flat.

An anabolic effect can also occur from eating medium-rare and
rare prime rib beef. So maybe it has something to do with eating
raw animal food. Everyone knows that medium-rare steak is great
for bodybuilding and muscle growth.

So support your raw milk farmers. I once paid $54 for 3 gallons of raw milk, $8.99 per half gallon x6=$53.94. Not only will you get raw casein and whey proteins, calcium and magnesium, your essential major minerals, hydration, good bacteria, no bad bacteria, but you'll be shifting the marketplace from bad to good, dirty to clean, man's ways to God's ways.

And if you live in a state or country that outlaws raw milk, then educate your government officials, and if they won't listen, team up with your local organic dairy and buy a portion of a cow, and as co-owner of the cow, you are free to drink its milk raw.

The issue is Clean milk vs Dirty milk, not Raw vs Pasteurized.

ABC Water and the Number Crunch Diet
Alkalinity, the untold secret to health and energy.

12 Changes A Year
Build a NCD Recipe Repertoire

Volume One
When you take control of the numbers you take control of your weight.

Volume Two
Begin today and forever be in control of the numbers you're eating.

Volume Three
You have to crunch the numbers to see what you're really eating.

GOOD Bacteria – your other bodypart
Looking deeper into your body's 2nd brain.

NCD Lactose Intolerance Protocol™
Number Crunch Diet method to Wean Yourself Back on to Milk

NCD Emergency Meal™
one quart of 2% milk

Recipe makes 8
3 items
1. 1 gallon whole raw milk
2. 2 half-gallons skim raw milk = 1 gallon
3. 10 grams of nonfat powdered/dry milk, x8=80g total

To a 32oz bottle or jar, see photo at the bottom of the homepage at www.abcwaterandthenumbercrunchdiet.com, add 16oz 486g of whole milk, place the jar on the scale, turn it on, pour in 486g. Zero the scale by pressing "tare" and add 10g of dry milk. Zero the scale, press tare, and add 16oz 490g raw skim milk. Cap and mix, refrigerate. Repeat 7 more times. You now have 8 liquid meals.

Tip. Dry milk spoils quickly, so you must consume these within 3 days. To extend the expiration, top the bottle to the brim with water so there's no air, then cap it. Or omit the dry milk, that's fine as well. The raw milk I buy doesn't 'go bad' it just gets better.

The Numbers are:
Calories = 495
Fat Calories = 140
Saturated Fat – not an issue on the NCD, (within range/limits)
Cholesterol – not a "bad guy" anymore, (or haven't you heard)
Sodium = 464mg – it's from natural sources, not added sodium
Carbs = 221 calories
Fiber = 0 – have a NCD Calorie-Free Vegetable later on
Sugar = 213 – drink it over 30-45-60 minutes to slow the release
Protein = 126 calories
Percent macros are 45% carbs 29% fat 26% protein.
Calcium = 1300mg – your RDA and then some
32oz of liquid (hydration with minerals)
$3.03 per serving
No need for probiotic supplementation – this is probiotics.
All gastrointestinal function – perfect!
Have half, 16oz, for a 250-calorie snack!

Some of you may be thinking, 16 weight ounces is 454 grams. True. The gallon of milk weighs 3977g, the empty jug and cap weigh 89g, so the milk weighs 3977-89=3888g divide by 8 = 486g per serving. The skim milk was a bit more, 490g. A gallon is 128 volume ounces, divided by 8 = 16oz per serving.

You're becoming a Number Crunch Expert already.

Page 276 ABC NCD

The raw milk dairy that I purchase milk from is called Organic Pastures, and you can read about the safety and health benefits of raw milk at their website www.organicpastures.com.[1]

They even have an annual "Camping with the Cows" customer-appreciation event, where you can take your kids and a tent and sleep outdoors, learn about organic farming, and take part in the quart-of-milk-chugging contest. How fun is that!! I betcha I could win! So support your local raw milk farmers.

Jumper Publications and Media

For the people who don't need a placebo-controlled, randomized, crossover, double-blind scientific study.

But instead, look to their Divine Intelligence for their reference.

The next time you hear someone say, "I got rid of my XYZ health problem by cutting out milk," ask them:

Well what kind of milk were you drinking?

---

[1] JPM and the author have no affiliations with and have not received financial compensation of any kind from Organic Pastures Dairy.

ADD-ON

In 2005 I read the book *Dead Doctors Don't Lie* by Dr. Joel Wallach. It says on the front of the book, 40-million audio tapes distributed worldwide. I listened to the cassette that came in the mail, bought the book, read it, studied it, and came to understand the importance of major minerals, minor mineral, and trace minerals. If you don't have time to read it, just take a high-quality Coral Calcium supplement. Open a capsule and sprinkle it on your food, your oatmeal, mashed potatoes, on a salad, and do it with breakfast, lunch and dinner, one capsule per meal, 3 per day.

Dr. Clark Store is the leader in purity, and so be sure you buy a pure supplement product, www.drclarkstore.com.

Anyway, Dr. Wallach is in the public domain again, and he is still preaching 92 essential nutrients. Nutrition and nutrients are key, as your body makes cells from what you give it or fail to give it. Dr. Wallach is also big on eggs. Also good advice. However, he never mentions milk, and actually shies away from it. As a farm kid and a Veterinarian and a Naturopathic Doctor, I would think he would preach milk, but if you sell a mineral supplement, then you wouldn't want to promote the drinking of milk (since milk is liquid minerals).

This book never addressed eggs, as it was about *Raw Milk*, but eggs and milk go together. Both are great foods to be eating, and the raw-er the better. In *12 Changes A Year, Volume 3*, I have a recipe for eggnog with a raw egg. It's numerically perfect, and tastes just right.

Lastly, the Flax Council of Canada and WebMD websites state that King Charlemagne passed a law that you had to eat flax seeds. This was 1250 years ago. You know that your body cannot "make" minerals, so you have to eat them. But you need to think of omega-3 in the same way, you cannot make omega-3, so you have to eat it, and the correct way, *NCD Flaxseed Shake Recipe*. Jumper Publications – the not bought-and-paid-for Science & Research.

PREVIEW
from the
ABC Water and the Number Crunch Diet

As you know, the recipes for the NCD are being published under the titles, *12 Changes a Year* – the companion guide to the Number Crunch Diet. It may take up to a year to get them written as it will comprise about three volumes. In the meantime, you can get your pH paper testing set up and determine your current alkaline stores. The recipes read like a book and include additional information that I've discovered about diet, lifestyle, health and selfcare. I look forward to seeing you over there!

To join my mission in providing people with safe, effective, affordable, selfcare protocols, send someone you know to www.abcwaterandthenumbercrunchdiet.com. Tell them to take the Quiz!! Thanks for your support! God Bless.

Jumper Publications & Media
From Advice to Results

I almost forgot! (again, not really) to tell you!

If you liked this shake recipe be sure to check out

TCY
12 Changes a Year
Vol 2

for the NCD ORANGE SHAKE!
It makes 9, and I often repeat the recipe midweek.
And whey protein – but not from powder.

BUY THE BOOK!!
IT'S GOOD STUFF!

Leave a Review

Without giving away the contents, "spoilers", recommend this publication and leave a review so that someone else might benefit from it too. Thank you.

www.amazon.com   Search: Raw Milk common-sense

Subscribe to my YouTube Channel
www.youtube.com   Search: Number Crunch Diet

Be sure to send me an email so I can periodically keep in touch with updates and new Selfcare Strategies – and discount offers on new items (yes, more than books!) (a simple and effective weight-loss device) (a weightlifting "device" that I use EVERY time I work out) and don't forget the recipes! – TCY.

abcwaterandthenumbercrunchdiet@mail.com
Privacy – your email address will not be used for anything other than by Jumper Publications and Media.

Saliva vs Urine pH

Top Ten Reasons Why Saliva pH Is Worthless When Compared To Urine pH For Acid-Base Analysis

#10 Small Volume – small tiny volume samples don't represent the whole

#9 Difficult to Obtain – the procedure is to bring up saliva and swallow, 2x, then use the third one for the test, too hard to obtain

#8 Poor Reproducibility – when you retest your saliva sample, you will likely get a slightly different color (reading)

#7 Poor Accuracy – if you collect a second sample, it will likely give you a different reading than the first

#6 Bacterial Contamination – bacteria from your mouth will interfere with the test

#5 Food Contamination – food from your mouth will interfere with the test

#4 Spoon Contamination – the surface of the spoon that you collect it on is going to affect your small sample

#3 Viscosity – saliva is too thick and results in faded or dual colors of the test pad (or paper)

#2 Difficulty Reading – the color doesn't "lock in" so you can take a reading, it tends to change shades through a range

#1 Your Salivary Glands have ZERO to do with Acid-Base regulation. Try Kidneys.

Your kidneys are running your body's alkaline status.

And your alkaline status is the secret they don't want you to know.

JPM Oral Hygiene Protocol

This publication is the introduction to JPM. If you paid $2.99 for the kindle version or $4.99 for the paperback version, then you basically paid for the two protocols, the xxxxxxxxxxxxxxxxxx, and the Secret Weapon, xxxxxxxxx gum-line cleaner. You will notice advertising for the other publications. Don't be upset. You got your $3-5 worth. The same cost as for a venti mocha latte, that's long since gone. The information in this publication will be with you for you to use for the rest of your life, every day.

So, why not take the ABC NCD Quiz!

The first half of the book is all about alkalinity. The secret aspect to your health no one, but a few, will talk about. However, no one covers the subject better and more comprehensively than in ABC Water™. The second half is the Number Crunch Diet™. No recipes, but lots of good sound information on diet. You will learn a lot, as no one discusses it the way I do. I brag a bit about the book, because it's really a great book. It's a compilation of nearly 100 books that I've read. But more of a Synergy, a new approach.

The recipes can be found in *12 Changes A Year* and you can see a sample on www.abcwaterandthenumbercrunchdiet.com

The title *Nontoxic Teeth Whitening and Dental Hygiene System* begins with the two chapters you just read, but includes a one-of-a-kind food-grade teeth whitening system, if you feel you need more whitening. It also includes a commentary on fluoride. Wouldn't you like to know if fluoride's something you should be doing, or something you shouldn't be doing?

So put your thinking cap on and let's start the Quiz!

It's good for you!

Pick the correct answers – There may be more than one

1. A urine pH of 5 is telling you
   a. about your blood pressure
   b. that you're tired
   c. about your alkaline reserves
   d. to see a doctor
   e. that you're healthy and fine

2. Urine pH testing is routinely performed by licensed
   a. social workers
   b. clinical laboratory scientists
   c. respiratory therapists
   d. fitness advisors
   e. nurses and doctors

3. The cost of one month of urine pH testing is _____ the cost of open heart surgery (CABG).
   a. 1/10
   b. 1/100
   c. 1/1000
   d. 1/10,000
   e. 1/100,000

4. The opposite of metabolic acid is dietary
   a. phosphates – found in meats and cola drinks
   b. bicarbonate – found in packaged foods
   c. caffeine – found in green tea
   d. bicarbonate – found in fruits and vegetables
   e. bicarbonate – found in oils and fats

5. Information can be of which types
   a. true
   b. incomplete

c. false
d. clouded
e. secret

6. "Natural Flavor" on a food label is
   a. natural flavor extracts from plants and fruit
   b. glutamates, MSG, altered salts
   c. chemicals that make you addicted to the product
   d. generally safe and good for me
   e. not something I need to worry about

7. During World War II, the people who failed to act early
   a. suffered
   b. died
   c. lost everything
   d. became victims
   e. made it through unscathed

8. Compensating means
   a. saving for retirement
   b. eating foods that lift your mood
   c. doing something to mask something
   d. brushing it out of your thoughts
   e. pleasing others and being a do-gooder
   f. all of the above

9. The reason(s) people are fat
   a. they're born that way
   b. they don't make their own meals
   c. hereditary – handed down from your parents
   d. my body just won't lose fat
   e. they don't see the numbers in what they're eating

10. The "Cheat Day" is
   a. a great way to get food cravings satisfied
   b. required to reset my fat-burning hormones
   c. a 2-8 step backwards day
   d. works well for most people long term
   e. is a popular "trick" that you should buy into

ANSWERS

1. A urine pH of 5 is telling you
   a. about your blood pressure – No, but there is a relationship (see Chapter 24)
   b. that you're tired – No, but there is a relationship (see Chapter 20)
   c. about your alkaline reserves – YES! Get to know your alkaline status by reading this book.
   d. to see a doctor – No, but it can lead to that.
   e. that you're healthy and fine – One number tells you little, 35 numbers a week tells you a lot. Get to know your urine pH.

2. Urine pH testing is routinely performed by licensed
   a. social workers – no
   b. clinical laboratory scientists – Yes, 99% of all urine testing is done by a CLS.
   c. respiratory therapists – no
   d. fitness advisors – no
   e. nurses and doctors – Doctors do perform urine tests in their offices, but they are not looking at urine pH with much depth.

3. The cost of one month of urine pH testing is _____ the cost of open heart surgery (CABG)(a bypass, "cabbage").
   a. 1/10 – no
   b. 1/100 – no
   c. 1/1000 – no
   d. 1/10,000 – Yes. You can test all of your urinations for about

$1 a month (see Chapter 11). A cabbage would run you at least $10,000.
   e. 1/100,000 – no. But I believe the potential to save yourself $100,000 in medical treatments is very possible.

4. The opposite of metabolic acid is dietary
   a. phosphates – no, phosphates contribute to acidity
   b. bicarbonate – no, bicarbonate yes, but not from packaged foods
   c. caffeine – no, caffeine is a drug, most drugs are acidic
   d. bicarbonate found in fruits and vegetables – Yes!
   e. bicarbonate found in oils and fats – no, oils and fats are not sources of bicarbonate

5. Information can be of which types
   a. true – Yes, this is a bit what your life is all about. Finding the truth about things.
   b. incomplete – aka, partial truths or half truths, aka, "spin". Do you find your head spinning when you go for fancy medical treatments?
   c. false – lies, yes lies. Don't call them untruths. Lies are Lies. When people lie it's your job to call them on it. Otherwise, "ya got no backbone".
   d. clouded – blurry, muddied, confusion. I could write "scientifically" but I would just make you confused and half lost. How does that help you.
   e. secret – Now we're talking. When they say "buy this stock" you've got to be a moron to buy it. The payoffs and the winners are kept secret, shared through word of mouth.

6. "Natural Flavor" on a food label is
   a. natural flavor extracts from plants and fruit – Well, they would like you to think that, but that's far from reality.
   b. glutamates, MSG, altered salts – Yes, often this is the case.
   c. chemicals that make you addicted to the product – Yes

Absolutely
d. generally safe and good for me – don't buy that line
e. not something I need to worry about – you make your own choices in life

7. During World War II, the people that failed to act early
Referring to this is grim and bleak. But there are people suffering and dying every day because they failed to act early. You could say that WWII is still happening all around us in the United States of America today. My book can help you not to fall victim to this death and suffering. So that you make it through your life, unscathed.

8. Compensating means
   a. saving for retirement – no, but I have seen people who are just a little too attached to their portfolios, compensating?
   b. eating foods that lift your mood – no, but food is commonly used to compensate
   c. doing something to mask something – Ah-Ha, Yes.
   d. brushing it out of your thoughts – no. It's okay and healthy to let go of thoughts, just be sure you're not avoiding your issues.
   e. people pleasing – reward seekers may be compensating
   f. all of the above – no, just C. Go back and read C again.

9. The reason(s) people are fat
   a. they're born that way – don't give me that
   b. they don't make their own meals – Bingo! This is key.
   c. heredity – your fat jeans are because of your fat genes – no I don't think so
   d. my body just won't lose fat – I hear you. There is not a lot of good help out there. Luckily, you've found the right place.
   e. they don't see the numbers in what they're eating – Yes. And person D above just needs to look at food mathematically (and read the book).

10. The "Cheat Day" is
   a. a great way to get food cravings satisfied – Wrong. I'm a testimony of getting rid of food cravings. See Chapter 38, 39, 40, 41.
   b. required to reset my fat-burning hormones – Wrong. If you get your macros right, your hormones will cooperate just fine.
   c. a 2-8 step backwards day – On page 84 of *The Four Hour Body* the person states that he gains 4.4 lbs on his cheat day. Then he loses it. Can you say "moody"?
   d. works well for most people long term – After reading dozens of diet books, I could not find one that worked long term, so I made my own. It's called the Number Crunch Diet.
   e. a popular "trick" that you should buy into – The Number Crunch Diet isn't about cheating. Although it's full of useful "tricks" that I came up with and use daily.

You'll be miles ahead of the average person after a while.